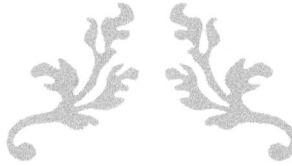

THE TALES OF TWO CITIES WHAT WAS-WHAT IS

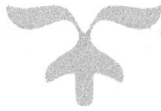

Gwen D. Rutledge

ISBN:978-0-578-63032-8

Dedication

Through my journey of discovering who I am, as I have evolved into the second phase of my life. I must say it was challenging and an awakening for the most part. During my search of me, myself and I. I learned a few key things which were patience and never stop learning. You never know where your journey and thoughts will align. I would like to thank my entire family, My Husband, my rock, Rodrick Rutledge who I love and cherish daily, for all his support. To my son Raghib and my daughters Hattisha, Roderica, and Erica. My granddaughters Razayia, Rhianna and grandson Jyhmir along with our 3 beautiful great granddaughters Jali'anna, Nova and Nyaila. And my sisters Lisa and Net. The road has been rocky with all of them at times but we managed to pull through. To my loved ones who have moved on into eternal life, some of their passing's created the will and determination for me to continue. Heavenly thanks to Grandma Fannie, Brother-n-law Henry Rutledge Jr., James Williams (Wax) and a special acknowledgement to my daughter-n-law Lashanda Anderson. They all were so special to me and will never be forgotten! I would like to thank my Pastor Rev. Dr. Alyn E. Waller of the Enon Tabernacle Baptist Church and my entire church family for their extended support and inspiration that they just couldn't imagine. I thank you all dearly. Last and so important my dear parents my Mother Sharon H. Spady and my father the late Nathaniel Spady, without them I would not be here. I will always cherish the memories and life lessons that you both bestowed upon me and shaped me into the woman I am today. Just understand and know that none of this could have been possible without all of you. I sincerely love and thank you all.

Acknowledgment

Dr. Christine Thorntup/ Dr. Wesley Muhammed

/Dr. Josh Axe

Coach Jesse Thompson/ Dr. Sebi /Dr. Namu

Dr. Bobby Price (Dr. Holistic) /Brother Rizza Islam

/Dr. Asu

Chef Ahki/ Sisters of the Macabee /Herbalist Kareem

(4 cycles of life)

We must do better in self-love; this is one of the first things that is required for caring for self before you can care for anyone else. You are a reflection on how you genuinely care about yourself.

Table of Contents

The Tales of
Two Cities What
Was What Is

Lesson 1

New Beginnings

Growing up as a little girl in the city of Philadelphia, was an awesome time as a child. I had no worries in the world and with being the middle child of three sisters, I was young enough to play on the block with my friends and old enough to be liking boys. This was such an awesome feeling back then, feeling grown and as the elders would say smelling myself. Just imagine, during these fun times as an adolescent, running up and down the streets and having friends near and far; playing games like catch a girl-get a girl and of course hide and seek, our it games.

During this era of growing up, family structure and discipline was in full effect. It was normal for 2-parent households to exist back then, sadly to say, unlike today, it seems to be the impossible. During my upbringing, certain conditions permitted us a family to have productive structural systems designed and created by our parents. This became a domino effect that has worked for our family as well as many other families during this time. First and foremost, we had to go to school which was very important to us as well as our parents. After a full day of school, we would return home to change out of our school clothes; then complete our homework and proceed to our scheduled chores. And then the fun starts; going outside to play was our reward.

Then once 6pm approached we would return back home for the family dinner and you betta not be late! Or there was going to be a price to pay. Now, once we adhered to our designated curfew times, we were able to go back outdoors until it started getting dark or 900 pm. whichever came first. Then prepared for the next day to do it all over again. Our parents didn't allow any foolishness or take any mess, this routine was typical for all our families. We continued to do this schedule until we entered high school. Now back then, during those years, when evening time approached, dinner time was important to us as a family. After playing outside with friends and conversing over food during dinner.

The importance of a good home cooked meal was something to look forward to. During this time, it was such a common factor for all of us to come together as a family. A typical dinner for our family was a meat, starch and a vegetable that was the normalcy for most families back then; it was all we knew. And during this time, we tried not to leave any stone unturned about our daily rituals. Because let me tell you; if my parents were to hear something good or bad that had transpired due to our behaviors; you would be in for a rude awakening! That definitely would've been a big problem. So, as my siblings and I would converse over our meals, we would always revert back to who is the best cook between our parents. This became a challenge for us, so they thought! My sisters and I would all yearn for the taste of our Mom and Dad's delicious cooking. My dad just knew he was the best cook that ever did it. My dad would cook for the most part, when he was in the mood. There were times we became skeptical when my dad would cook, we never knew what we were eating until his concoction was completed.

And boy were we in for a surprise, I'm just saying! he would fix dishes on special occasions like rabbit and deer and then try to disguise it as chicken or something else. As you can see, my mom didn't cook as much but her cooking was just as tasty and delicious. Now I must say, as I reflect back during my younger years not knowing each night what the food selection would be, it was like flipping a coin guessing who got it right for dinner! Our parents also allowed us to utilize the kitchen to share in the lessons of cooking. Both of my parent's techniques of cooking were different but very important, my dad was more adventurous my mom was more basic. On the other hand, my mom really loved when my dad would cook. My mom didn't have the desire to cook much, but she loved being waited on at all times, and who wouldn't. Now, at this time we were able to learn about various techniques such as frying, baking, steaming and boiling while preparing meals. Here is a glimpse of some of the food choices that became a staple in our home and most family's homes during my years growing up. These were the foods we lived by then and for some even to this day.

It was all parts of the chicken even down to the gizzards, so many parts of the pig, pig feet, pig ears, ham, pork ribs and chitlins which were the intestines of the pig, lamb chops, all parts of the turkey, oxtails and last but not least beef, steaks of different cuts and ribs. And of course, we cannot forget the vegetables, collard greens, string beans, black-eyed peas, sweet potatoes, yummy potato salad, corn, white rice and the mandatory dish is that scrumptious mac n cheese we couldn't live without. Now to top it off, white bread and cornbread yes, we had to have our bread. I know you have to say to yourself Dammann we as a community were eating and still eating all those animals and starches like it's the last day on earth. Mind you, my sisters and I didn't indulge in many of the various meat choices; we thought it was so gross, seeing the actual body parts of an animal and then devour it. Now, what was so important to us as a whole, was being altogether as a family during dinner. We would reflect over each one's day while enjoying family conversations and giving everyone the opportunity to vent or receive clarity on their views.

Each topic of discussion at the dinner table became the entertainment for the evening. Now, as you can see, during the early stages of our cooking experiences, we've learned, retained and acquired the knowledge at hand. So, with that being said, we now have basic skill sets to become self-sufficient to utilize when needed. This exposure has allowed my siblings and I to explore and experience many types of food. Even during my years in school, the school system played an intricate roll with explaining guidelines of nutrition with the food pyramid by way of teaching and understanding the dynamics of good health. There were health classes, that explained the do's and don'ts of good nutrition. School teachers would teach and grade the fundamentals of nutrition and all that it does for the body.

Those poster boards of the infamous food pyramid / basic food groups were our guide. These poster boards were embedded for us to envision truth and facts and then bestowed upon us as students to adhere to policies on the how, what and why of understanding nutrition. This also aligned with the same nutrition techniques that most families endured then and even now.

Mind you, the majority of health practitioners and nutritionists would share these same views, standing by the relevance and importance of this now known culprit! Now, with all due respect, at the end of the day cooking became less interesting and the streets were becoming more intriguing and fun! My focus was having fun and being cool, that was all I wanted to do at the time. And boy, did we have fun, my favorite saying was let the games begin my friends! So, as I continue to flourish while living my young adult life, it has had its challenges. Everything was becoming fast paced as I was becoming more independent. And yes, during this time the powers at hand were slowly encroaching their version of good health on us as a society. They continuously shoved this thing called the standardized diet / basic food group down our throats. And now, we have realized it has created so much havoc on our health, which I didn't discover until much later.

So, let's dig into this thing called the basic food groups / food pyramid which represents the standardized diet. The food pyramid/ standardized diet was considered significant, this format of nutrition was advertised and put on display in health classrooms, nurse and doctor offices and facilities that aid in any health practices. There were poster boards displays of dairy-meats-grains and carbohydrates. This pyramid, was created in published in Sweden in 1974. Then in 1992 the USDA [United States Department of Agriculture] followed suit and that is when the pyramid was created and established and dictated to us as a society in these yet United States. Now let's elaborate on these food groups! Meat-with all due respect is derived from living, breathing functional animals that produces and give birth to offspring's in similarity to humans. These animals' functions within their own world and habitat. Continuously they are preyed upon, slaughtered and consumed for human consumption.

Some animals are treated and cared for in a cleaner and healthier environment other are mistreated, degraded beyond recognition and held in the most horrific conditions. Even still, no matter the process they have organs that are aligned to work and function as human beings, such as a heart, eyes, noses, mouths. These animal voices will wale to no end at the hands of their killers screaming to their vocal cords collapse fighting with the last bit of strength and breath left in their windpipes from their helpless turned lifeless bodies fighting to survive. This process is inhumane! All for the selfless intent of humans salivating their so called acquired taste. So, doing my quest of understanding the standardized diet. In the summer of 2017, there was a buzz going around about a Netflix Documentary called What the Health. This documentary had everyone talking and becoming more aware of what was going on within the food industry. It sparked a reaction with people from all walks of life, everyone had something to say! This information was an eye opener; which caused a whirlwind of reactions.

Some people became more aware by wanting to make changes within their diet, food choices and overall health. Then you had some die-hard believers that believe there is truly nothing wrong within the food industry such as the nutrition, labeling etc. Through the many facets of confusion of people's reaction, it led to a worldwide quest to reveal the results of the documentary What the Health by another documentary called Vegan 2017 that can be viewed on

YouTube. This information became so instrumental while understanding the foods we eat. So, during my seek and search, I came across a man by the name of Dr. Sebi, so many revelations had transpired from listening to his documentaries and speeches. Now I can see some of the cause and effect within our food. I can truly say this is when I's are dotted and the T's are being crossed. Dr. Sebi was a man with a vision to save the world and reveal truths to the American Diet. His beliefs aligned with other scholars such as Chef Ahki, and Dr. Holistic who also admired the works of Dr. Sebi and understood the misconceptions of what we were taught pertaining to eating meat, poultry and even fish.

They would reveal the false reality of what nutrition you, we, thought would be gained from eating meat such as protein and zinc etc. the truth is, you can receive these same nutrients from plants and vegetables. Studies have shown eating meat can cause and does more harm and damage to the human body more than you know, such as high blood pressure, heart attacks, strokes, kidney disease, liver disease and the list goes on and on. Then we have: Dairy-The biggest culprit I know is this mind clogging, blocking, hardening to the digestive tract is dairy. We really are addicted to damn near all dairy products such as different assortments of cheese, milk, yogurt, mayonnaise and butters this I must say was challenging and as I stated before it's hard as hell, yes addictive but you must make the changes. It will make a world of difference for your health and to your health.

Then we are told that we need milk for calcium to enrich our bones how about it's been documented repeatedly that milk deteriorates our bones and health faster than anything else, this poison should be removed from markets, stores and wherever else it's sold, it has no nutritional value what's so ever! It is a benefit for the calves the cow's babies just like our milk the woman's breast milk should always and only be consumed by our babies point blank period. As an alternative I would like to introduce you all to what I consider to be the most nutritional milk, hemp seed milk, hemp seed milk gives so much more nutrition for babies as well as adults. And then there's the: Carbohydrates- Now, some may say what are carbohydrates? Well there is fructose, glucose, lactose and starches. We specifically want to address the refined carbs. Which are found in foods that are such as your white pasta, rice, bread, starchy vegetables, grains, pastries and cereals.

Here is another untold truth about this 5-letter hazard that we call carbs! There is a danger of having too much refined carbs in the body and the result can become dangerous which can lead to someone having a host of all sorts of sickness and illnesses. We must understand, the body breaks down or convert some of the carbohydrates into sugar glucose which is absorbed into the bloodstream. We, especially as indigenous people, we need to focus more on ancient grains and sprouted type foods when it comes to our pastas, breads, cereals etc. Ancient grains and ancient grain products are originated from its natural state and sources it is considered GODS food. Ancient grains, have been around for centuries and holds the highest nutritional value for us as well as our families. Whenever you want to purchase any type of carbs source of food seek out ancient grains and sprouted foods you would not be disappointed! Last but not least, we have: Fruits- How sweet it is! fruits that is, the only thing to be said about this topic, ONLY EAT SEEDED FRUIT! PERIOD! Now, to be totally honest the USDA have continuously played a significant position with our nutrition for at least a century.

Starting from the 1916's, even until now and over the years the name has changed on many occasions for this so-called food pyramid. Now with so much information on how to eat healthy, this food pyramid was all designed for young children to get the best nutrition. Prime example: Everyone simply assumed the food pyramid was like a bible guide for healthy food, if you did not consume your foods by this format it was considered you were not eating healthy. These 4 food groups were designed and created to sustain good health for a healthy lifestyle and this so-called food pyramid came at a price. Which may leave us to wonder why so many people have no clue of what is truly going on with our food and all the culprits involved. At the end of the day, when it's all said and done, food has taken us all on a journey, we live and learn and continue on the good, bad and indifferent of challenges that it brings.

Lesson 2

Quick-Draw-ma Draw:

Now lets' visit the 80's and 90's era, during that time period, I was matured as an adult and times were changing, moving fast and our foods were definitely changing for the worse; microwaves were taking over! This time for real and at an alarming rate. The history of this quick machinery was developed and produced after World War 2. It suffered and lacked the design structure and sizing over the years. From 1946 to the late 1970's the microwave had many challenges from various companies to meet the needs of the consumer.

The 80's and 90's is where the microwave became a staple and necessity to the American people. This is when everything fast was in full effect during this era everything was in quick demand, from living on my own to the food you ate. And yes, the fast food industry became such big business during this era. Everyone was moving quick and experiencing the got to have it right here moment!

This became the traditional way of cooking for most families and fast food restaurants had become the dinner table for most, along with the in & out methods of the drive-throughs. The thing that is so sad to the got to have it right now era, if I could be honest, we really could have done without it. It was basically wanting and not needing. It became an addiction for the majority of us, it was fast easy and yes so damn tasty too. I'm not going to lie I know it's a hard thing to give up! But we must look at the big picture overtime of the long-term damage and effects occurring to our bodies from this got to have it right now era. Here is a snap your finger example, how the fast foods became readily to purchase at such a low cost, I mean very inexpensive, available for kids to even purchase. These different food items were being priced very low and ranging from only $2 and up-not exceeding $5.00, then came the $1.00 menus that had no thought process at all. Just readily and available to purchase, consume and damage the body.

Now, can you imagine overtime the magnitude of destruction that lies dormant awaiting triggers that will set off explosive stages of destruction; causing detrimental disaster to the body, is absurd and no one ever thinks about it! And yes, we {USA} continue to fall victim to this quick fix, microwave diet preparatory habit of eating. With the high demand of wanting it right now. This urgency has created the food industry to meet and deliver in such alarming rates. Which then led most of the food industry to create dangerous ways to process their foods for these demands. So, now when the microwave era started encroaching upon the early 2000's, no one was listening or paying attention to our children's health this became the risk factor of the fast food industry's success. No one had a clue of the rapid rate of the risks and demands that brought upon the dangers on families from the fast food industries.

Then in the mid-2000's, our First Lady Michelle Obama, who stepped in and stepped up! on children's obesity, she took on the biggest issues and concerns dealing with obesity. This was at the forefront of her agenda the children of our nation became her first priority to learn about the foods that we all eat by way of understanding limitations and the importance of being active. It was a home run and created change within schools and homes across the United States. Everyone was jumping on board during Michelle Obama's quest to fight childhood obesity. There became a health craze wave that creeped up in every state, city, community and most importantly schools.

Michelle Obama enforced the food industry to clearly display additional product information on the labeling of their products. And this was the time for everyone to understand the language on what was being put out into the market. Yes, it was an awesome got to have moment to have such a powerful woman of her caliber; making such a huge mark in the food industry it simplifies that someone cares.

Now, with all that being said, I guess you may ask was I a victim of those quick fix meals during the quick fix era? Well of course, I indulged many times going through drive-thru restaurants as well as sitting in fast food joints. Enjoying those same meals as some of you continue to do so, until this day.

But those moments did not last forever for me. Since I can remember for some unknown reason, I had adapted a consciousness of healthy eating. I created techniques to keep myself at a stable weight such as not purchasing clothing in larger sizes. Once I reached a comfortable weight it became my anchor of stability. As an adult this tool became my guide even to this day. It allows me to adjust when I'm heavy or even losing weight just by the maintaining of the fit. I always say, never buy larger; this has become my rule! thee rule! Another was, don't do too much of anything such as drinking of alcohol, snacking or digesting meat on a regular basis. The biggie was no sugary drinks, I was never a fan of sugary drinks. This quick fast microwave era continued to bring its challenges for some. Have you ever wondered how did we get here with food? Food! Food! Food! Yes, it's very delicious and addictive, it brings comfort to all and it's a way of gathering people for a cause, reason or a function. Food is a necessity for survival.

Some people can go 100% indulging in food to their death; then you have some that utilize strategic methods of indulgence in their food. Then the food industry has gotten to the point of let's just satisfy everybody at any cost and that is exactly what they conspired to do. It seems as though they hold a philosophy of, If, they are going to eat it we are going to make sure we will have it, readily and available. Let's just give them what they want and when they want it!! Now did parents know better? well, I would say yes and no for the most part because most of us lacked education and knowledge on healthy foods. Majority of us have been misled about a healthy diet, you can only trust what you prepare in your own kitchen for your children with the right information, with that being said of course everything is a gamble when trusting strangers within food establishments with our everyday food consumption. At the end of the day, you really have to be the judge, jury, prosecutor with a clear mindset of strategies from the beginnings [intake [to the ends [digestion] when it comes to your health.

Lesson 3

SUPERSIZING

SUPER SIZING, is where the microwave era leads us with food as well as our body images. Our body image changed drastically from indulging in the supersizing of our foods to super-sized body images. This may have lead individuals from one extreme of self-medicating with food to not loving themselves or for whatever reasons that would place them in a state of depression, sadness or full scope of anxiety. This has been one form of sickness or disease that may have caused some individuals to seek surgeries to address obesity. Remember, it may not be addressing the underlying issues that even gotten an individual to that point to even have surgery. On the other extreme sometimes food or the trickery of what food can do may have triggered one's mindsets with feelings by any means necessary to go under the knife for a nip or tuck altering and improving their body images, when there is nothing to change for some.

This has become a normalcy in our society just like purchasing a cup of coffee every morning from a Dunkin Donuts or Starbucks. As you and I both know going under the knife is just a quick fix. Cosmetic surgery is just a surface enhancer just as cosmetic make-up. For some a little nip and tuck can be just fine for some but in reality, you must apply a maintenance regime for the long haul for your overall physical and mental stability of good health. You must be true to yourself, for that daily or weekly regime, it should become a staple in an individual's life who seeks out these types of surgeries. it must be for the long haul. At the end of the day, always find personal time for yourself and self-reflect, there is nothing in this world greater than having calm and peace within, you have to demand it for yourself. If you don't take care of you then who??? This all goes back to the saying you are what you eat? True or False? Well over the years, so many of us discovered that all truths on eating "healthy" has been in question. We've learned that our diet has implicated changes on our health through the years that brought about changes within history.

From being bamboozled on the standardized diet to a compromised artificial diet to the chemically imbalanced diet. Now the standardized diet and pyramid guide has proven to be especially unnecessary for indigenous people. Keep in mind, anything that's standard for everyone should be in question. There is no way the word standard should and could be standard for all people, due to qualifying factors such as genetics, culture and the list goes on. Now again, we were told about the food pyramid which consists of dairy-meats-grains-and carbohydrates these 4 food groups were created to sustain good health and a healthy lifestyle. This thing called the standardized basic food group has created havoc on indigenous people. For those of you who are not familiar with the term indigenous people, they are known as the first people, aboriginal peoples or native peoples. They are ethnic groups who are the original settlers of a given region. Indigenous people are totally different by way of culture, food, beliefs etc. which is a very important component to us as a people. We have to first understand who we are as a people and not get caught in the bamboozled trap listening to others and not seeking your own truths.

Prime example, some of us still don't embrace breastfeeding some think it's a disgrace to nourish our own because of being uncomfortable of it all. Then we ridicule our own if the child stays breastfed for too long. When in fact they were getting the best of the best nourishment that is genetically and Godly for their digestive systems to contribute in their well-being of good health. Yes, it's horrible how we don't take the time to understand our bodies along with good health, which goes back to the inception of life. We must understand we have always been a people of resilience, strength, patience, nurturing and compassion even to our enemies. We have always been misunderstood and considered people of discovery for them. Now as we know the American diet / soul-food we considered it to be our own, by default, our ancestors became the creators. They became so creative, they made their cuisine from the masses at hand, their garbage. Their seconds which were leftovers [slop] became a meal we call today, our soul-food.

And yes, it became perfected over the years and very tasty too. With that scrumptious taste of soul food later some of it came with all sorts of additives, GMO's, you name it, it's in it and that's where part of the death of our destruction begins. Thru this history as we come to know this soul-food, it became a course of bad health. Even to this day it is very hard for us as indigenous people to understand the depths of destruction it has upon us. The meat, starches, sweets etc. Years ago, some parts of the food of the soul food was in good standards, grown with no preservatives, no GMO [genetically modified organisms]. Since times has fast forward to quick fixes, it became the root and because that crippled us with so many illnesses, sickness and diseases which plagued us as a society. The hurt and harm our bodies endured from this soul-food diet became damaging to our health over the years. The question becomes can it be modified to be prepared healthier? Well of course it can! As I will share later. Being raised off of soul food early in life & now we are fighting for our lives! This is the part that we brought upon ourselves from lack of knowledge.

We have been conditioned to think old programming and never adjusting or changing channels to improve our mindset for a healthier lifestyle is the norm. If we simply just take a few steps back and debunk most of the information told to us on how to eat and live and inspire to live a fine luxury lifestyle by way of spiritual, mental and physical we would become greater as individuals but also stronger and wiser as a people. What I have learned is to educate! educate! Educate myself as well as others. This is something that our communities are seriously lacking. To understand the needs and functions of the body we must seek and find the truth to all our questions which is right at our fingertips. The problem is that we don't want change, change is needed for the good of our souls. So many people have issues with new things. There are rewards and consequences to everything you do, you must pick a side! We as a people struggle with doing what's required. Why is that? we don't even know. That brings me to something, I Call an ah ha moment. What I would like to refer people to is a book called who moved the cheese, some may be familiar with this book it has been around for years. Who Moved The Cheese is very enlightening on adjusting to life challenges?

It is even relevant till this day, when I was one sided on the wrong track of things not wanting change from a previous job. The Executive of the company introduced this intriguing book to me it was an easy read. It helped me align my thoughts and put everything in perspective. When you find yourself at a crossroad this book, Who Moved The Cheese became that learning tool I needed to get back on track. Cleansing your mind, body and spirit is another component to getting mental clarity it's one of the many things I utilize to clear my head space from overall negative energy. With that being said, your diet is key, it plays a significant role in healing the body it could either nourish you or kill you. That's why seeking natural sources are a must. Some of us are unaware of GODS natural supply. I became an avid listener of Kareem the herbalist, Dr. Josh Axe, Sisters of the Maccabee as well as Tim Morrow who share in the holistic version of healing.

There are so many natural herbs that heals the body. I'd had first hand experiences that I live by. Just to name a few that is a staple regime for myself as well as my family. Herbal / medicinal Teas-Dandelion, horsetail tea, hibiscus tea, ginger tea and moringa tea, sarsaparilla tea, green tea and nettle leaf tea just to name a few. I do not proclaim to be a doctor nor am I a doctor but I can say this from my experiences, all these teas and oils have medicinal properties and from my experience they work! All of the teas aid in lowering your high blood pressure

- Horse-tail-specializes in hair and nail growth, oral hygiene, diuretic, strengthens bones and tendons etc.
- Dandelion-detoxifying, builds immune system, high in antioxidants minerals & vitamins etc.
- Sarsaparilla-anti-inflammatory, arthritis, protects the liver, cleanse the blood, aids in the cleansing of mercury in the body etc.
- Hibiscus-major effect of lowering high blood pressure, boots liver health, weight loss, lowers blood fat levels etc.

- Moringa-fights free radicals, fights inflammation, supports brain health, protects cardiovascular system etc.
- Ginger-relieves nausea, reduces inflammation, fights respiratory problems, strengthens immunity, relieves stress, etc.
- Nettle Leaf-may treat enlarged prostate systems, may aid blood sugar control, may reduce inflammation, supports eye health etc.
- Turmeric & Ginger-strengthens the brain with functionality, memory reduces inflammation in the body, boost your immune system, cleanse digestive tract, removes plaque from arteries etc.
- Sea moss and Bladder-wreck-The powerhouse of them all. Has 92 minerals for the body. It is the electricity that sparks everything within the body, from your joints to cognitive function. Literally a cure all for any and everything within the body!!

Cooking Oils:

- Grapeseed oil-used for cooking especially can be used in high heat
- Coconut oil-can be used for cooking as well as on the body to heal, soothe and oil body.

Medicinal Oils:

- Oregano Oil-improves gut health help treat yeast infections, treats fungal infections, heals wounds, fights bacteria, helps lower cholesterol etc.

Frankincense Oil-opens your chakra for spiritual awareness, heals wounds and scars, may reduce arthritis, maintain oral health, may fight certain cancer, immune system, improves digestion etc.

Cayenne Pepper-natural blood thinner, helps for smooth blood flow throughout the body, prevents clotting. Some herbs I utilize such as-cilantro, basil, smoked paprika, rosemary, all-purpose seasoning [I utilize these most of the time when cooking]. All organic. At the end of the day, you are what you eat and a true manifestation of who and what you can become, take care of you because you are all you got!!

Lesson 4

Sea Saw Confusion:

Yes, taking care of you should be a priority! some may, some may not, but sometimes life has a way of showing you if your slacking or just need to tighten up. I've always been someone looking for the most natural holistic way of centering my life and utilizing the oils as stated above. I find it so rewarding to share this information with the world. For those who may or may not know is all I want to do is try to make another individuals life much easier and happier, now to confirm the effect of these herbs and oils, I want to take you guys back in time a little bit, let me share a little story with you guys, just stay with me. Approximately in the month of February, the year was 2015, while the radio was playing on a pretty fair weather Mid-afternoon, I was upstairs in my bedroom, just took a break from trying to straighten out my bedroom closet, I had so many things going on in my head from getting ready for this girls trip, to things I needed to tackle when I return.

This has always been my world of crazy, always trying to do a million and one things at a time. I'm sitting on my bed; I then get a phone call from one of my nieces. My niece and I started going over preparation for our upcoming girls' trip to Las Vegas in March. This trip included my daughter, 4 nieces and 2 of their friends. The processing for this trip was fun but also exhausting, from making sure I can satisfy everyone wants and needs within a certain price range. So, as my niece and I finalized somethings we then said good-bye and I then go back to straightening the clothes in my closet; basically, trying to analyze my wardrobe for our exciting girls' trip. My husband then enters the room and says you still working on that closet? you going to be all day. I replied "no I'm not, I just got off the phone with our niece, Terry, we were going over some details of the trip". Within seconds, as I was standing by my nightstand, I had a strange feeling that came over me, not sure what it felt like, but I sort of felt light-headed and I just kind of tried to ignore it.

I then said to my Husband Rod, 'babe, I'm feeling kind of funny' he then jokes around like he usually does and says 'you probably can't go on your trip' I then laughed and said.

'oh yes I Am you know I'm going"! And boy, my husband knows how I love to travel. Rod then turns around and goes back downstairs to finish cleaning his car in the garage. Then a few minutes goes by and I'm still feeling strange for some unknown reason and I started saying to myself, what is going on? then I paused for a second and said to myself I'm okay, I'm okay, I'm fine. Then I continued to keep doing what I was doing putting my things in place. I then drank a glass of water that was on the nightstand. As I began to drink the water a weird intense strange feeling came over me as though I was present but not present, if that makes any sense. So I decided to slip something on then proceeded downstairs pass my husband, saying to him in the garage I feel so weird, so I just got into my car and told him as I was leaving, 'I'm going to the emergency room', he's looking at me not fully understanding what I'm saying or where I'm going.

As I'm pulling out of the garage, in that split second you would think we were in a silent movie with no sound. I knew I had to just go! While I'm driving, the only thing I could think to do and knew how to do was pray. But I'm going to keep it real, this praying time was different, I was praying for the person driving which was me but didn't feel like me. So, I arrived at the hospital, which was approximately 10 minutes away from our home. The intake nurse started processing me, I'm sitting there in a daze. She takes my vitals and my pressure is through the roof 240/150 OUTRAGEOUSLY HIGH!! The intake nurse says Oh My God, do you have HIGH BLOOD PRESSURE! I replied no. So, they rushed to get me a room and started hooking me up with everything, asking all these questions pertaining to any sickness, illness or diseases and I answered no to everything. My husband arrives with fright all over his face, not knowing what to expect and each doctor that entered the room spoke to me repeatedly asking if I had HIGH BLOOD PRESSURE, I repeatedly answered NO!

So then, they asked all the normal things of family history and any medications. I was then informed that I would have to stay overnight which led to a 2-night stay. They wanted to run all necessary tests to rule out any and everything they could think of. They came back with their only findings is high blood pressure. Now, during the day of my release they gave me a prescription and I was told the norm to follow up with my primary physician. So of course, Rod was there to pick me up. Once I came home, Rod asked how was I feeling since I was back home, I said, damn this so messed up! Rod started laughing, then I started laughing, before we could even sit down, we were looking at each other like this can't be real, we know is not a laughing matter but we were laughing, Rod said un, uh that old age setting in, Rod always mess with me about the age saying. If you know me, I always said, don't claim old because you would start feeling old and being old.

I told him; I was definitely still in shock over the scare I endured with my health thou. But hey, what are you going to do? Rod couldn't believe they were saying I had high blood pressure. Shoot, I couldn't believe they were saying I had high blood pressure! I know, I know, you probably saying what's the big deal? Just about everybody has it. What you guys don't understand, we try to live a pretty clean, healthy and productive way of life. We eventually made a few jokes about it, discussing all the limitations and stigmas attached to high blood pressure. But then I went into my undefeated space! I started saying oh, no, I'm not going to be on no damn pills! I'm going to beat this thing! Yup this is how we challenge each other to do our due diligence and be greater than before. Then I just started thinking out loud, like damn, I Never really been seriously ill only a common cold here or there and a little problem with my sinuses that would flare up from time to time. Then Rod just looked at me and we just started laughing out loud again. If you guys knew my husband, I tell you no lies, I really think he missed his calling as a comedian.

Now here we go, so my husband accompanied me to see my primary Dr. I explained everything to her in reference to my episode at the emergency room and their diagnosis of me having high blood pressure. She takes my vitals; my pressure was a little abnormal not much but my doctor goes over all the things that could cause your pressure to soar. Well of course, your diet, weight gain, stress and sometimes other health issues. She says, you know you're going to have to change something. I'm looking at her like what is she talking about? I really wasn't trying to comprehend what she was saying because I felt like I had not done anything different. As you can see, I'm still in denial. I looked towards my husband and said "this got to be some cracking bull crap," you should have seen me, I started doing a quick flashback trying to find what did I do wrong. I practically said to my Dr. "I really don't eat a lot of bad stuff." If you could have been a fly on the wall. I was spasming, as though I was on trial like I committed a murder or something. I Just could not wrap my head around taking pills, medication, prescription drugs or whatever you want to call it.

So, I went into defense mode explaining what I ate then and what I eat now. I started rambling on saying I don't eat too much junk; I love sour cream and onion chips and some pastries here and there. I told her I don't drink sodas, sugary juices, not even orange juice. I do eat pork ribs maybe 2x a year and a cheesesteak once a year so sparingly, I do the gym every so often. Rod was like snap out of it, during that moment I paused and caught myself didn't even realize I couldn't stop talking, I was going on and on, Rod said, "you just have to get more strict and Really watch your salt intake" my Dr. was in alignment. I actually felt like they were double teaming me for a minute, I'm just saying". At that point, I was on board to do whatever was needed for me to live a healthy and productive life and lifestyle even more so. So, a few weeks went by and you all know I still had my girls trip on my mind but still not understanding why my pressure had me feel that way; with a sense of urgency and need to go to the emergency room the way I did, I was still baffled.

I'm going to say this, I never ever felt so weird and strange in my life and scared as hell not knowing the known or the unknown of my health. And of course, I did comply with what my doctor required of me to continue to take the pills. Well the show must go on, right? We here baby, now this can't be hard, while here in Vegas, I'm going to do what it do, you feel me! I'm watching what I eat not indulging or applying any salt on my food this has been the norm for me anyway. I told my daughter; I'm still feeling a little funny here and there but it comes and goes. For the most part I feel okay, plus my daughter Tisha can utilize her nursing skills, so I'm good, booyah! So now we are feeling ourselves on some grown and sexy fun. Always being careful and aware of my intake as well as what I'm feeling and I remember my doctor saying it may take some time for the pills to get into my system. So, I kept that in the back of my mind and continue to have fun on this trip in Vegas baby!!! And that's exactly what I did, I continued to have an awesome time in Vegas.

So, as the trip ends and we are EnRoute back home to the cold, I realized that trip was so necessary. I think everyone should travel to warm climates in the winter, especially people of color, one reason is, we become so depleted of vitamin D, I'm just saying! Now here we go, a month or so goes by and I have to make a visit to my doctor because I'm still not feeling like myself. Mind you, I was trying to adjust to this concept that I would have to take these BP pills (blood pressure). So, during my visit, of course I explained how the pills are not working, my doctor insists that I'm not giving the pills enough time to get into my system. My pressure goes down for the most part. Then my Dr. and I go back and forth as though we are playing a game of tug or war. It seems like a battle, trying to get her to understand what I was feeling. As I tried to explain to her the feeling of overheating and not feeling like myself and my pressure keeps fluctuating going up and down. She was still insisting the timeline of the pills. Trust me I get it, but what point do your Dr. honor what you say, even though I know she means well.

Then she hit me with the willie bobo, and goes over my age as though Rod was talking threw her. I could 've wrung her neck playing the age card! And that's not all, she put the nail in the coffin she mentioned the C word, for you guys that don't know that means the change of life. You know what I said, "I already know of my change of life, I'm aware. Now, we are playing baseball, my turn. So, Doc, what you're not understanding when I experienced the hot flashes prior to all this blood pressure mess, my flashes were bearable but since taking these pills it seems to bring them on even more and I don't understand why. Well after she heard me complain over and over again, she changed my prescription and says, 'when you take these give it some time everything should adjust', I said "okay". Swoooo, Dammann, I felt like I had to run to every base for that! Please yawl, don't judge me, but I don't want to take these damn pills. Only because I still had a hard time wrapping my brain around taking medications, I know in my heart of hearts it's something else causing the elevations to my pressure; I have not done or been doing anything drastic that would have caused this change.

But of course, as we all do, I followed my doctors' orders and started taking the BP pills again, since the dosage had been increased just a little. When I first started taking the second set of pills, my head was pounding like somebody just took some screws and tried to twist them in my brain to look like Herman the monster! baby, those pills made my head feel like a truck ran over my brain. After about 3 days the pressure subsided and I took the pills for about 2-3 weeks again. See, what I went through, that's what pisses me off and that's the reason why I'm not keen on taking meds they always make you feel jacked up. After sometime as in a few weeks, the same feeling of overheating, lightheadedness and not feeling like myself. Those same changes had occurred again. Mannn, this was becoming such a pain in the you know what! I started googling about the BP pills. I went so hard during this ordeal to really make a change or a difference whatever you want to call it. I wanted to make sure I did everything right, such as my food intake changing drastically, when I say my diet changed!

It really went to almost nothing; I wasn't eating much or putting salt on anything. I constantly checked my sodium intake with foods that had a lot of sodium in them, like ketchup and many more common everyday foods. I lost so much weight and didn't even realize it. Family that was around me every day didn't see it but others had noticed the change. But in all, I still didn't feel any better just not feeling like myself. So of course, constantly talking with my husband and my immediate family about the frustrations I was feeling; I started wondering if it was depression, then I was like no, that's not it. I started thinking it had to be something else, no one could understand what I was feeling, it, seems like we as a people always have to put a name to something to identify it. I knew whatever this was it was not going to defeat me and I was going to get to the bottom of it no matter how long it took. You can't put a price on happiness, and yes, I went on each and every day working my job dealing with people and their crap with a smile on my face. Even, dealing with my family and all that entails as though I was okay and everything around me was fine but at the same time, I felt withdrawn at times.

I didn't really want to socialize with others as much, I just felt like, life was zapped out of me mentally. I know some of you may say and title it as depression but I didn't think so, I know you guys wondering how did I know? Well, I had some experience or should I say symptoms that I've been thru back then in the mid 80's when I felt like I was at a low period in my life due to other life changing circumstances; That's a whole other topic. But doing that time being focused on GOD and having my Grandfather by my side, that's all I needed, I was good! So, let's stay focused err body, lol! Let's fast forward, I had to go back to my Dr. to inform her that these pills were not doing me any justice, I insisted that something else was causing my pressure to keep going up and it wasn't due to my weight or the food I ate. I went through all of that with working out and daily monitoring of my food intake, yes, the weight came down; and still issues. My Dr. made a point to me, she said "do you want to live"? "or do you want to die"? I had realized in that very moment; this was something that caused me to really wrestle with.

Not so much of the yes or no answer if I wanted to live or die. But more so, if not taking of these pills will determine my faith. Something was truly wrong and this isn't the answer for my pressure it's definitely something else. I told my Dr. I wasn't trying to be difficult but again the pills seem to be causing more of a negative reaction than anything else. Ok, so I told her I would take the pills, mind you, now I had like 3 different bottles of them. I left her office with the mindset and determination that something got to give and it isn't those damn pills. I always challenge myself to get the best results for myself. Just a note to all, I don't recommend anyone not to listen to their Dr. but what I do recommend is for you to do your due diligence for your health and yourself. SOOO, what I discovered remember, the conversation about the C word and age. As I researched low and behold thru the process of elimination, what I discovered was. I was going thru bouts of anxiety. I was feeling overwhelmed, getting older worrying about the next chapter in my life and started to feel like a worry wart always worrying about my family as a whole and individually, as well as loved ones and close friends.

The truth about menopause, it can teach you how to relive life or it can take you on a mental collapse if you do not get control of it! More likely than not, menopause was the underline issue of all of the above. It causes and triggers a lot of things in the woman's body. And one of them is anxiety. Anxiety makes you feel like you revved up, moving too fast, over thinking everything and racing thoughts etc. always rushing, extreme thoughts on the what if and no peace and calm in your life. So now, the challenge is what do I do to get things back on track. First you have to slow down and stay in the moment. Breathing, deep breathing that is. It is such an important technique it rejuvenates your cells. So many women such as myself, have a lot on our plates. I spoke with a sister friend of mines, low and behold she shared all the same symptoms and signs that was pointing towards high blood pressure.

I encouraged her to share the same information with her doctor to break down what I discovered to see if her Dr. can address her situation from the angle of anxiety. Well of course she didn't follow through, she was afraid to do what was necessary to change. So, she continues to take the medication, I truly understand it's hard to create your own lane. What I've learned is that some will and some won't and it's okay. We as women, carry the world on our shoulders and wear our hearts on our sleeves; so yes, as I stated previously, we have to take time for ourselves, by utilizing deep breathing techniques and finding peace within every second of time. I believe if we as individuals wanting to make healthy choices, we need to apply these things with the proper diet. I'm going to put a pen right there-to discuss the term 'Proper Diet `"quote un quote" this became confusing when I thought I was doing the right thing at the time of the BP discovery. Oh, how wrong I was, I tell you know lie when I hear the saying learn as you go. I literally, was doing just that! I was experiencing so much on this journey of trying to do the right thing.

One of my scariest moments, when I thought death was knocking at my door, I didn't know the day or the hour. This is what I know, over a couple of days I was feeling like a cold was trying to creep in on me. So, this one night, I felt myself slipping into a head cold that then turned into a sinus infection that I periodically would get but this time I noticed after a few days the infection went away from taking an antibiotic but the cold stayed which didn't make sense to me. I then started experiencing an uncontrollable cough at night that had become very scary! So, I made another appointment for my primary Dr. as an emergency visit. I was prescribed a cough syrup for my cough, as the days passed, I continued to feel horrible my cough turned into a strangling uncomfortable cough with leakage going back and forth to the bathroom mainly at night while sleeping. Then during the day, I would leak every time I coughed which became unbearable to be at work at times. This had now started to affect my day to day activities nothing was working.

I literally was falling apart and my breathing was being affected 100% I felt completely like death was near because there was no answer to my illness or what was going on and nothing was working, I was totally out of answers. I returned to my Dr. again demanding answers to this madness and I was not leaving until there was an answer for this death like experience. We talked in length from my hour to hour to my day to day activities and regime. I was so zapped and drained. From the coughing, losing my wind of breathing to the leaking and constant changing of clothes throughout my days. We then discovered through conversation that my cooking of onions and garlic smothered over my food which became the ah ah moment my Dr. explained they are acidic (garlic and onions). My Dr. recommends that I would need to start using an inhaler he stated I was experiencing a form of COPD (chronic obstructive pulmonary disease) or acid flux-GERD (gastroesophageal reflux disease).

Well, I assured my Dr. I am not using any inhalers, once I refused the inhalers, I knew changes had to be made and I would do whatever it took to be back to myself again. There wasn't much left to say but for me to make it happen. I then went over my diet and made adjustments. So, I knew the change would take time but I was still dealing with the strangling cough, leakage and not being able to sleep at night I was totally exhausted. I still needed help so while EnRoute home, I searched high and low for an ENT specialist in my area. Unfortunately, it was the same office I visited a few months prior when I experienced another ENT who wanted to do surgery on my sinuses which has always been an issue for me. Once I did my research on the medical terms used for the one day, procedure I then realized my issue was minor for the sinus surgery, of course I cancelled; go figure! That was my fear of getting the same specialist in the same office.

Now, the next ENT Specialist within the same office I was able to share my symptoms of the strangling cough and leakage she knew exactly what was going on. I was overjoyed and said Praise GOD! The ENT Specialist stated I was experiencing silent reflux where there is no heartburn or feeling of acid rising in the throat it clearly all happens in the back of the throat. She prescribed a steroid along with something to take at night to help me sleep. I asked how long would I have to take the medication she answered it could be a life time or not long at all, she said it all depends on me and my diet. Some people take anti-acid tablets for this just to enjoy their foods when in fact just tweaking a few things with your diet is all you need. Those tablets eventually burn your stomach lining and damage your organs with long-term use. When I tell you, I slept like a baby, OMG, I was in 7th heaven. Well I was able to get my first good night sleep that night then from there I was clear within a week from everything. I thank GOD for her knowledge and experience. Yes, I dove into learning more about what foods to eat and what foods were acidic forming. I definitely do not eat garlic anymore and only organic red onions. Since these changes I've been able to breathe and resume back to my life as I knew it.

Now back to our previous conversation of the proper diet and getting rid of the meat, dairy and processed foods also continuing the use of medicinal teas is priceless, with that being said, I knew, I would be just fine. Every doctor visit since the discovery of these revelations from changing my diet had been a success. With techniques like slowing down, getting plenty of rest, exercise and not rushing all the time and having patience and I can't forget that me time! Another key component I have discovered is that going to bed approximately between 1030 pm-1100 pm is crucial. During this time, your body actually goes to work to stabilize and regulate your hormones also when persons go to bed late you can never replace any lost sleep. Another tip is not eating from 4am-12pm this is the cleansing cycle-detox, flushing the lymphatic system at this time allows your body to reset. From 12pm-7pm is the intake cycle- your time to indulge in eating meals.

You must also feed the body high nutrients and drink plenty of water at this time. From then 7pm-4am is the assimilation cycle-digestion and rest the intestines all are so important. With that being said, I will continue to seek natural health alternatives and resources for the good of myself and others while finding and creating quality time. At the end of the day, no more pills! your girl was able to conquer all the above, you and only you can change your life course, never settle for less, always fight to the end for a better you and what you believe!

Lesson 5

Menopause Monopoly:

So, now women and gents, here is what you all need to know, that when it comes to the understanding of this thing called menopause, most women and majority of men have no clue of the effect it has on the women's body. You must understand and be aware of all that it entails. You will never be able to cope with life in general of all that is to come, so with that being said, If, you do not mind, I would like to expand and ponder on the C word or change of life if you will. This is one of those things that can be crucial to life or death. I would like to share or enlighten those who may have been experiencing some of the following trials and tribulations relating to menopausal symptoms.

Before I was able to pinpoint the cause and effect of my own episodes with prescriptions drugs for my high blood pressure I was still unraveling and trying to understand the levels of menopause, these issues were happening simultaneously, not to mention I have been dealing with fibroid tumors since I became premenopausal. For those of you who are not aware of fibroids, they are benign tumors that grow from muscle tissue in the uterus. These tumors can enlarge profusely and cause excess bleeding months at a time, severe pain in the abdominal area and it can become so unbearable at times that some women have been encouraged by their doctors to pursue a hysterectomy for relief. It's so crazy, that now if truth be told, hysterectomies should never have been a go to for any woman. There is so much information out there now. Your primary diet is your form of medicine.

Just to inform you, when it came to my fibroids each doctor's visit with my gyn Dr. she would monitor my fibroids, they would enlarge at times then she would inform me that they would show shrinkage at times. She never understood why was that but that was good news for me. I must say, I felt like I was on a crazy roller coaster ride with the different challenges my body has been taking me through. During this time, I was approximately in my late 40s-early 50s, everything was copacetic, I mean, I was living my best life. I was encroaching upon my entrepreneurial skills as a high fashion jewelry consultant to becoming an Independent jeweler in my own right and named it Fine-Luxury-Living. I was living in the moment and experiencing what I called the good life, feeling myself and enjoying my family at the same damn time. Traveling and meeting a lot of influential people, I was doing the damn thang. I was working on branding and venturing into other business ventures.

Through all of this, I started creating an indecisive space of unsurety. Didn't know how or why this was happening but it was. I said to myself "self, what the hell is going on"? Of course, I had no answers, lol! but my mood and mood swings were slowly becoming annoying. As I would Interact with people that were close to me, such as my family, I was becoming more difficult to converse with at times. My attitude was so flighty just like my moods, wishy washy! It had gotten to the point my husband became just as agitated. My behavior was becoming horrible with just regular conversations. And after each mood swing of loud talking, defending attitude and my irritability I knew I had to get a grip. Every time, I looked back on my behaviors I'm like wow! The flashbacks were real, my children didn't even want to say much to me not knowing what they would get in return. I was so embarrassed not believing that I was actually responding in that manner.

If you guys would have seen me, it was not a pretty site. Talk about mood swings, OMG! So, of course, I knew something had to be wrong. So, when I attended my gyn Drs. appointment, I couldn't wait to discuss the matter at hand. I discussed everything with my doctor and I was already aware that I was going through menopause. My doctor did a few tests and low and behold she said "I was smack dead in my menopause, It sounded like a bull ride challenge, I was being faced with, either I was going to go for the ride and hold freak-en tight or I was going to just fall off give up and wave the white flag! Of course, guys, I said to myself, not me! You should know by now I'm taking it to the limit. I'm going to ride that sucker like there was no tomorrow! I said to that damn menopause you're not going to beat me! I refuse to give up now I'm here to the wheels fall off! Then as I refocused, I was like, WOW FOR REAL! But wait a minute doc., then I asked, now I'm wondering what's going to be the next change if any? She replied, "the same but maybe more intense" I was like it is what it is! I continued to experience hot flashes as I stated before, mood swings were the issue. So that was my next question, my doctor explained no more or less will happen.

She asked if I wanted a prescription to handle my mood swings or if I was having painful sex and of course I said 'no'. I didn't need anything as always. All my routine doctors know I did not like taking any medications, but of course they have to ask. I still need to understand what is actually happening within my body while I'm dealing with this menopausal change. I needed to first get to the root of understanding what is menopause? As I read many articles it states, menopause is actually the beginning of the end and the coming of new beginnings as we call it the C word or change of life, cause and effect'. This is when the woman is at her pivotal age which is key! The woman's menstrual cycle comes to an end after one year of hormonal changes. It marks the end of the reproductive cycle and the ovaries decreases in estrogen production. I also was aware of the effects of menopause can be detrimental to your health, especially if you don't understand the process. One thing I know for sure is that your hormones becomes so out of control and that is the challenge. So, as I tried to seek out some answers about menopause, I came across many symptoms and causes that can affect the imbalances of change related to menopause.

From what you eat such as sugary foods, stress, which all can spiral into bouts of anxiety or even the effect of alcohol consumption which brings on the hot flashes and experiencing low moods once alcohol wears off. I was like wow, really. Now here we are back to the diet again. I can't stress this enough how our food is such a collation to you and your health. It's said that the same don'ts for high blood pressure also applies to the don'ts for menopause and fibroid tumors go figure! Which tells us that we as women let alone people have to get down to the nitty gritty of your health. Again, here are more of the red flags to look for: GMO labels, non-organic, pesticides etc. We are in a time now where buying organic, non-GMO foods and foods free of pesticides is so needed. That was the connection why my fibroids kept shrinking it was all due to my diet of eating healthier foods.

One day I was watching the breakfast club, a show that I watch on a daily basis it consists of 3 individuals DJ Envy, Angela Ye and Charlamagne Tha God who interacts with individuals by way of interviewing with many facets of people ranging from politicians, multitude of entertainers and everyday people who are making a difference. I later discovered during one episode of the breakfast club show there were 3 persons speaking on the topic of fibroids, Coach Jesse Thompson, Dr. Amun & Dr. Asu spoke in the depth of fibroids and endometriosis. That answered the majority if not all my questions. I was ecstatic that their it was, the root, cause and effect and results as I expected! All right there. It is so unbelievable, that when you can be grasping at thin air for a period of time then miraculously out of pure determination of listening to your body and gut feeling to know you are on the right path. To have confirmation to your beliefs such an awesome feeling you're doing exactly what you are supposed to do is be true to yourself.

Remember, there can be physical and mental changes to your everyday functions if you're not careful. These signs and symptoms can seriously affect you if you're not knowledgeable or if it goes untreated. You can treat it naturally or by your physician but you must pay attention to the signs! As I endured some of the newer changes that became somewhat intense and astonishing to me. I never had to consider any of this before. I said to myself, it's time to lace up my boots and get serious as I bark upon this journey of the big C. My philosophy has always been GOD always, in his infinite way, has the last and final say over everything. I always say, you should never ever settle. Make sure you get the best results, when it comes to yourself, needs and wants. And by doing that, there should be other resources to address our life changes as we mature and become older and wiser women, in this thing called life. As I experience another ah ha moment, one day I was watching an episode on Oprah Network called Super Soul Sunday. I came across a guest named Dr. Christiane Northrup who speaks on women's issues, she was discussing with Oprah about her dealings with menopause and menopausal symptoms like most women go through during this crucial time of the unknown.

I was so pleased to hear this conversation, because some women treat it like a disease, or the unspoken word. One statement she said that made a lot of sense. 'Once woman reached this pivotal moment in their life, which is the 2nd half of their life. It is a time to reflect over your life and re-evaluate all things to come for the future. A light bulb went off. Duh! I was like OMG! It's official, here it is loud and clear. The confirmation of it all, I can truly see this being the reason for the unsurety of what's to come in my life. Dr. Northrup states this period is when all your goals, desires, dreams is at this time in our life on what are you going to do about it. As women we have a tendency to look so far ahead and even to our deaths to assure everything would be taken care of as we would want it. And during this time, the bottom line is you either poop or get off the pot. Your tolerance levels are very limited you can't deal with much nonsense anymore or bull-crap! Again, this is when you're working on the second half of your life; Being focused and living your best life is key! I said this is exactly most of my thoughts, on life and my tolerance of things, so of course I retrieved her book from the library and wow it was a lot to read and I dove in.

This gave me a whole other perspective of understanding this process on a medical and technical standpoint which was great. During this process everything was starting to become clear to me, I knew I wasn't the only person or woman going thru these changes like this. So, I went on a mission and starting talking to my elders, seniors and loved ones as well as my friends, trying to get some answers. So, while visiting my mother, I would ask how did she deal with her coming into her change of life, she stated she basically would just try to stay cool by putting cool cloths on her at times. I also remember during our family gatherings which we had a lot of. My grandmother, Moma as we called her and my Aunt Verna and of course my Mom, would be sitting in the dining room sipping and shooting the breeze and playing their oldies that I loved so much. When I tell you, when I walked in the house it looked as though they all would be running a race on who could fan the most that's what it looked like walking into that room. I thought it was crazy to see that! I remember saying oh no! "I don't ever want to go through that, damn, you guys that hot"! and they replied we are having our own private summer and you going to get to experience it too. I was like oh no I'm not and left them sipping and fanning away.

Then we have my mother-n-law Nola, I sat down and approached her with the same question. If she could tell me what did she use or take to deal with her menopause. At first she was tickled and just smiled, she said she would always eat a lot of ice and instructed me to do the same to see if it works for me, she then said 'it always worked for her and that's all she ever did, "so just eat a lot of ice baby." And yes, I asked my friends mothers and basically, they stated the same thing over and over again about hot flashes. Of course, I asked my friends they didn't even want to express or share no more than the hot flashes. I was like you know what, everybody walking around saying to each other, "I don't want any negativity around me", or "I can't be bothered" here's another one "I just stay to myself" oh and we can't forget I just need peace of mind I stay in my lane, I have a lot on my plate and I can't handle any extra drama! I realized all that was doing is telling me that they too were going through some changes but not acknowledging climate change. At the end of the day, as women we were all saying the same thing. It seems to me that women were afraid to share and reveal what they couldn't explain when it came to the change of life.

I was so confused and not understanding how do we as women can't even share our physical or mental changes of ourselves that may help the next sister. That is just so strange to me. I was like damn, so I came to the conclusion that our elders and my fellow sisters really didn't understand or even had a clue about what was going on in their bodies or what they're bodies were even going thru. As you can see again, the collation of my episodes with BP, menopause, fibroid and Diet it all intertwines. There is much more to the human body, especially the women's anatomy. We are the breeders of human life. While understanding the importance of what you eat is crucial to bearing a life with capabilities of sustaining oneself. As we move forward and continue to enlighten those who are still unaware of the movement for a clean environment and healthy lifestyle, they too will be at the forefront sooner than later.

In the movie Forrest Gump he says, "life is like a box of chocolates" and I would add, life is also a present-as you unwrap it, you would have to unpackage your peace and happiness with clear understanding of having meaningful relationships. This will represent the present, and the gift of life that you can share and give to others with meaning to enjoy this fine luxury living lifestyle. So, I am here for my sisters whenever they need me! So, at the end of the day, I will continue to help, guide and provide individuals who are interested in taking their first step in making a difference for themselves.

Lesson 6

When You know Better, You Do Better:

As we continue on this journey of seeking out the truth and trying to be rid of sickness, illness and diseases. The search is never ending. Unraveling what's good for us and which foods can give us the best nutritional value to sustain good health definitely comes with challenges. We will continue to make the best choices for us as well as our family. With that being said, if there is anyone interested in taking steps to a new way of eating to live, I always say: Step 1- you must eliminate and remove all meat from your diet, which means pork, beef, chicken, rabbit, deer and duck. I guess you may be wondering why not fish? Well I figure getting rid of all those animals for some, may have you in a shock and not want to continue but you can have fish or any type of seafood which allows you to be now considered a pescatarian, what so many people find easier to transition to.

Step 2, is to eliminate all the dairy such as cheese, milk, mayonnaise, yogurt, butter and of course you must do away with eggs. What I found to be helpful is finding alternatives to your most common everyday go to foods such as your mayo, cheeses and butters. For those items veganese is a very good mayo go to, it doesn't contain any dairy, soy or eggs. For the exchange for your butter I use Miyoko's cultured organic vegan butter made from plants, it does not contain any soy or gluten. Follow your heart brand of cheeses which I use sparingly. These cheeses are very tasty. When it comes to milk, DO NOT use any type of cow's milk, not even 2%, and no soy milk. Some may think that almond milk is good, I guess it would be better than cow's milk. Coconut and walnut milk are a great choice but I find it to be too thin for me. I discovered hemp milk which is made from the hemp seed, very tasty it has a shelf life of at least 3-6 months or more and it's worth the purchase you can make your own hemp milk just purchase hemp seeds and add water with some agave or dates whichever you prefer blend then drink.

Step 3- Is to become more conscious and aware of processed or packaged foods, they are very dangerous to your health. They contain a lot of sodium and preservatives. Such as lunch meats, canned foods, foods ready to heat and eat. Step 4-The old saying, everything white isn't right! That pertains to white flour, white sugar, white rice and white bread. There are flours that are designed for us as indigenous people such as spelt flour, garbanzo flour just to name a few you won't be disappointed. Instead of sugar I use organic honey no substitutes or artificial sweeteners are a no-no, been there done that. When it comes to rice there are so many, you have red rice, black rice, red quinoa, wild rice and so on they are ancient grains as well as red pasta noodles and rice noodles. Breads only purchase ancient grain breads such as spelt bread, Ezekiel breads or Ezekiel wraps etc.

Step 5-Vegetables, you may eat all vegetables except, spinach, broccoli and orange carrots. It is your choice if you continue to use those vegetables just mentioned, I choose to use spring mix to take the place of spinach; those don't foods are hybrids which breaks down in the body and turns to sugar. Remember hybrids are man-made by way of 2 plants or things put together with starch for binding. Once the foods are digested the starch breaks down and turns to sugar which becomes detrimental to our overall health. Step 6-Fruits & Nuts, eat only seeded fruits-Brazil nuts, Walnuts, and sunflower and pumpkin seeds is what I prefer and coconut flakes, coconut oil is also a good source of collagen for brain health, there has been claims the source of coconut by digesting it aids in the decreasing of Alzheimer's and dementia. Now, speaking on brazil nuts, let me tell you how good GOD is. as we age, most women experience issues with their thyroid such as I. So, I made an appointment with an endocrinologist who stated she found 5 nodules on my thyroid and vitamin D levels were in the single digit! So, I had to return for a biopsy and check vitamin D levels again. Low and behold after taking Cod liver Oil by Carlson 2000 mg 2 tablespoon every day for 2 weeks my levels were restored amongst with eating a handful of brazil nuts several days of the week which aids in the natural treatment for thyroid and hormonal health. Now the biopsy showed the nodules were benign. Praise GOD Word of advice never remove any ORGANS!

Now, once you allow your body to flush, it should take at least 1-3 months maybe 4months whereas your body will be going through a severe flush and beware you will be going to the bathroom on a regular until your body adjusts and resets itself from the cleansing of the waste and toxins in your body. Now mind you, once you stabilize your diet, your bowel movements will become more regular each time you eat within 3-4 hours you should release. There are so many food choices available that you can indulge in while on your journey. Now, when it comes to your seafood if you have decided to become a pescatarian instead of going cold turkey of eliminating fish that's all good. When cooking seafood make sure you do not cook with olive oil, only use to drizzle olive oil over your foods once food is cooked. Also, I utilize 2-3 days a week not to consume seafood yes, I break from the seafood to indulge in plant-based foods such as all organic vegetables for those few days. Now, while cooking foods at a high heat, you can do with grapeseed oil or sesame seed oil it's able to sustain the extreme high temperatures in place of olive oil. Remember, don't be misled or assume you can't live healthier without meat or harmful GMO foods, sugary foods or damaging carbs simply not true. That is what this is all about eating natural foods as much as we can.

Good food and good health go hand and hand. If we really care about ourselves and loved ones, we would take a strong stand about what goes into our bodies. We can not only think about the outward of ourselves. Our interior is the spiritual force of what we represent in a Godly manner. The old saying whatever goes in definitely must come out. Just think for a moment whatever is seeping through your pores such as pus, odor, secretion and any bulging through the skin such as bumps and lumps remember, that is everything we digest on a daily basis. Will we slip up? maybe, maybe not! We may fall short of something small or unconsciously but going back to meat is something we should never allow ourselves to do the same with hybrid foods. I want as many people as possible to change and adapt a healthy lifestyle, I can't reiterate it enough. Remember, at the end of the day, there are so many outside sources that try to disturb or disrupt positive energy we all have to start somewhere for a better you that can produce a better us, don't be afraid, positivity always outweigh negativity let this be the beginning of a new day!

Lesson 7

The Web We Weave:

And the spiral begins, so when people say they are woke, what does that actually mean to you? Does it mean being uncomfortable because you can SEE the injustices and you want to make a difference? or Does it mean you can commit to something for the good of mankind because you are woken? Now on the other hand, can you actually see why it's so important for us as a whole to make a difference for positive outcomes! Why? Because the parties at hand can portray a world of division by giving power to negative forces that would create or continue the path of destruction to us as a community, society and even the world. My favorite line is not on my watch!!! So now the question becomes, if you are still eating meat with your truth and facts, how woke are you? And then there's so much more. So, now again, if you sincerely are considered woke, that implies you don't eat food that harms the body?

We also know there is a process and levels to becoming a clean eater but in actuality whatever your preference is such as pescatarian, vegetarian or vegan you are on the right path. I believe woke also applies to living outside of the matrix. The matrix is real! Also being woke applies to persons who can see and are not blinded by overloaded corrupted systems at hand who are trying to make a dollar out of .15 cents; literally by any means necessary here are a few of those conglomerate businesses!

- Food-Industry
- Big Pharma-Pharmaceutical Drugs
- Healthcare-Industry

All the above [F.B.H.] can totally work against you and not have your best interest at heart. what do I mean? As previously stated, when it comes to the diet or food intake, we must know the do's and don'ts of it good bad or indifferent.

Food is a necessity but there should be a common sense of good health. You must know that the world of today, has participants with hidden agendas which are aligned with the conglomerate businesses stated above. The known and the unknown continues to confirm and speculate some of the dangers of the food industry that has been webbed into hoops and loops and no one knows how to break loose. The carelessness and intentions of those who set out to bring harm willingly is horrendous to the American people, yes, you heard me right the American people, why is it that only in the USA, we have dangerous hazardous causing ingredients allowed in our foods that brings harm to our overall health. It's very hard to wrap our brains around the processing and packaging within the food industry allowing the injustices by these webbed conglomerate businesses have this type of control. And that's why it is so imperative to be or become more aware of the atrocities that has been allowed to plague us as citizens of these yet United States of America. Brother Wesley Muhammed and Brother Rizza Islam had shared their views on the upside-down comparisons on designed neighborhood markets.

This documented information as also been exposed by Michael Nutter the past Mayor of Philadelphia, on a televised program walking the streets of Philadelphia with an analytical team. They revealed the comparison and quality of resources from various neighborhoods. All parties have agreed one way or another on these same issues at hand. This information has repeatedly shared information of documented events and statistics of how we are labeled as poverty-stricken neighborhoods. With communities that have poor health statistics is by no means an accident. It's all strategically designed with Allterior motives. This type of designed landscape of foods, good and bad, some placed in vibrant marketable areas such as the good foods who they assume are for those better than so called civilized citizens with stability and structure and then you have on the other end of the spectrum the bad foods for those so called don't want to do nothing, low income, submissive, struggling citizens in these areas. These poverty-stricken areas have no access to a legitimate, qualifying standard supermarket within a 3-mile radius in the inter-cities such as North Philadelphia.

Prime example for those who lives near 22nd and Lehigh Ave. The only market in this radius is the Shop-Rite market, don't get me wrong that market is pretty good but it does lack much needed organic fruits and vegetables, the choices and options are very slim. So, I tried to understand what it takes to get a full-fledged operable market within that area with the bells and whistles like any other family-oriented neighborhoods. So, I contacted the office of Cindy Bass-City Council for the area. I spoke with Cindy Bass assistance Mr.

Keon Holmes and Mr. George Stevenson on two different occasions. Mr. Keon implied Super-markets has to want to become a resident within these areas in order to serve these areas. I was utterly surprised to hear those words It was then suggested that I should become responsible to cater to the elderly to transport them back and forth, my response was WOW are you kidding me? Then you have Mr. Stevenson who implied, they as the residents of the community can travel to 29th St. for the Save A Lot food Store. if you are a senior or reside near 22nd and Lehigh Ave. You will have to take public or private transportation. My concern is that there has always been a somewhat market at 22nd and Lehigh Ave. Markets has downgraded for the worst in this area when in fact living in these times year 2019, we are going backwards instead moving forward with resources.

Then Mr. Stevenson stated part of the process is residents being notified of new businesses coming into neighborhoods along with those businesses while going door to door to notify residents of what's coming into their neighborhood. This is something I as well as others in the area have been totally unaware of. Then it became a back and forth in the conversation if I attend neighborhood meetings or not? Which is neither here nor there. Mr. Stevenson went to different levels of who I need to point the finger at. I stated it's not just about me! This is about the neighborhood and meeting the needs of the people with fresh produce they can purchase on a daily basis. It's alarming to see seniors having to travel on buses, hacks Ubers and taxis just to even get to the Shop-Rite Super-Market located at Fox St. and Hunting-park Ave. And don't forget some of the transporting continued to be done by way of family members on a regular basis to acquire adequate healthy food for their families within their homes.

This is absurd! What are our politicians doing to aide in healthy resources for our neighborhoods? With all due respect, do they really think the Aldi's, Sava lots, Dollar chain stores is actually good nutrition? It's something which is better than nothing but still not good enough! We as a community have to do better and understand we are in a state of emergency for our health! So, with that being said, in the meantime, you must continue to make wise decisions in what you introduce to your body and digest within your body correctly, why? because it would become detrimental to your overall health. To make smart choices, do not let them win!!! Which brings me to BIG Pharma! Which follows bad food choices, this is nothing new, it always comes into play once you go against the grain-with bad food choices. You will be wreaking havoc on your body and digestive system. Big Pharma prescription, medications, DRUGS doesn't discriminate, it will find you and wear you out! This continues to be the consequences of bad decisions. We as consumers, parents even as individuals we put ourselves in harm's way, more times than none. We allow the unthinkable to happen. Such as the sickness, illnesses and diseases, they start to brew. I can't say that all the mishaps that occurs from having bad health is totally all our fault.

We actually put so much trust in our doctors and wholeheartedly believing that our doctors are doing us justice by having our best interest. Which may be true! Then there is that percentage of doctors who really could care less and put their patients' health on the back burner. It is a known fact that these behaviors do exist that's why there's so much money being made within the pharmaceutical Industry. It is documented that there is a war going on between Doctors, patients and pharmaceutical companies giving insight and negative effects of the statin drugs. For those who are not aware that statins are drugs prescribed by doctors to lower cholesterol levels in the blood. It has been stated by doctors by lowering the levels it would help prevent heart attacks and strokes and even a percentage can prevent death from heart disease.

There are trillions of dollars being made off these statin drugs and many prescription drugs at the expense of the American people. Why do I say this? It has been documented that statin drugs alone do more harm to the body than good. Also, it causes more side effects than you can imagine. I understand people are scared to die and that's where the trust of the physician comes in and what do we do, when they say you have to take this and we go right along and do as they say and take it, I get it! Without any questions, research or clear understanding of what those prescribed drugs will actually do. Then as time goes on, we look in the mirror and wonder what happened, so many of us have been there. We have no idea how to get back to our normal but the downfall within our health becomes our new normal. But does it have to be? once we receive that diagnosis, we should respect the order from our medical professional and investigate the terms, diagnosis and treatments.

Then we can go to the next level of resources that can be accompanied along with natural alternatives for a positive outcome to have a better you. I'm not saying not to take your medication or utilize prescription drugs, what I am saying, we can prevent a lot of the mishaps that comes along with long time use of prescription medicines. Example: when it comes to blood clotting, heart issues etc. some are not aware that something as little and minor as cayenne pepper ¼ glass of room temperature water with a few shakes of cayenne pepper, is a preventive measure it can do wonders for the body, heart and blood flow.

Which brings me to the discussion of the healthcare industry. This is the last stop on what I would like to call as their gravy train. When you look at the big picture it's almost an assembly line. From the food intake-prescription drugs-healthcare Industry [hospitals, nursing home]. The tracks, is where these things live such as dialysis, needles [diabetes], stints, wheelchairs Hospice etc. There are roadblocks and reasons why we can't move pass go.

Yes, it works, just like that, when we don't follow suit with educating ourselves on the good, the bad and ugly of our diet this is what happens, we become susceptible to that vicious train ride. Don't get on that train! Don't take that ride, find another source of transportation to help you travel through this thing called life. We have to do preventive measures and become more proactive. All this is possible with GOD'S will, faith, mercy and determination. When all else fails, from the perspective of the doctors when you receive those words, there is nothing else we can do for Mr. so-and so or Mrs. so-n-so or they may be taken home to be comfortable until they transition, now you know you're in trouble now! or are you really? When I hear that terminology, I equate that line to you only can go as far as you're allowed.

This can be due to the level of insurance coverage compensated for care some coverage barely covers a ¼ of resources and some can cover almost 90% then those individuals coverage will sustain them to it's all evaporated and they then they too will prepare to be released with the saying there's nothing else we can do said by doctors and medical professionals. Of course, there are some that may be aware of natural holistic healing but not many. As I know, GOD's work is just the beginning, this is the time of everything from GOD's natural creations and raw foods goes to work to heal the body! When our loved ones are told those cold words to be placed on hospice and let the ending process of life take effect. Families please listen!! The only thing I have to say is don't give up! If your loved ones are still allowed to take in water or maybe any type of nutrients, give it to them but this phase would be totally different. They must frequently be given water for dehydration you may use a product called thick-it, it helps prevent them from aspirating and it goes down slowly and easy for them only if they can utilize straws, spoons or cups.

Next if they can receive any nutrients in the form of liquid give them green drink concoctions such as kale, collards or spring-mixes for your green leafy vegetable you can add different types of fruit for flavor. These fruits aide in the healing for sickness, illness or diseases such as an apple, soursop, dragon fruit, blueberries, or raspberries. Your loved ones must stay hydrated and also give oil of oregano by way of mouth 3-4 small drops in a ½ glass of water swiss around then have them swallow or take in by way of straw. This can be taken day and night this helps fights off damaged cells affected by cancer it rebuilds and restore the cells. This oil of oregano is a powerhouse and no joke do not use more than 10 days consecutively. You should eventually see results within 2-3 months depending on deterioration of the body. Also, oil of oregano can be used to rub on body to penetrate muscles from soreness. Frankincense can also be used in small drops and rubbed together with coconut oil on the body for arthritis, soreness and pain. Utilizing the frankincense oil on the forehead and back of ears down towards neck [lymph nodes area] on both sides helps keep loved ones in a calming peaceful state of mind. This action also helps Alzheimer's and dementia individuals.

So, my question to you, can you change your mind set to continue to fulfill the goal of healing and nurturing your loved ones back to good health? If the answer is yes, then you're on your way just believe, remember, FAITH without WORKS is DEAD! So, you must believe to achieve and watch GOD go to work! Just to reiterate I am not a doctor nor do I profess to be one but I solely can speak and share on my truths. You know, I believe in speaking positivity into the atmosphere and the universe. I remember watching David Letterman documentary on Netflix. It was an interview with Kayne West, he said something that I thought was simple and corky but also profound. Kanye West says, "I don't like to use the word diet because it has the word die in it"; his preferable word was live-it which definitely makes since it's motivating and inspiring to live on. If we start to exchange the word diet for live-it, can you imagine how that transitional effect of words may become significant in so many people's lives just to be put into the atmosphere. I love live it; it sounds more lively lol! Its sole heartedly starts with us! You know, we have this one life, that is delicate and precious some take for granted. At the end of the day, we are blessed with another chance at life to assist, aide and support others by way of life experiences or just positive supports to aide in the well-being as human beings. We must just try to always do something!

Special thank you:

I would like to give a special thanks to Darlene Tilley. She is a phenomenal woman; I clearly remember June/ 2014 at her niece Nokia Grand Opening. Darlene greeted my daughter Tisha and I and during our conversation she made claims of a prophecy that I will be writing a book along with many other things. That alone stood out where as I couldn't for see but she did! Fastforward life happens and that little voice that we ignore sometimes was telling me sharing is caring. As I was half way thru this project it dawned on me the prophecy from Prophetess Darlene Tilley, all I could say is look at GOD! Sometimes GOD sends his angels to give us just a little sprinkle of his grace. Always be kind to those who cross your paths, stay humble and most importantly be true to yourself.

I sincerely thank you,

With love my sister

Reflections:

As I self-reflect, over my younger years of life it allowed me to take a few steps back to consume and indulge on improving behaviors while enhancing my beliefs. Since my 60 years (7/59) of life thus far. With goodwill of cheer, the impact of my confidence and performance trying to live a good life-of the good life! as a human-being, can become challenging at times. I never thought in a million years, we, this world would be demonstrating such a power, that would succumb to fighting for our lives from the foods we eat. We as a society, have a duty to care for one another that is reach one teach one because as I always say, you are me and I am you and we are one. And as you and I both know, there are individuals who claim to know it all. They may also profess it in a way that they're not living or breathing it. Me personally, I do not profess to know it all or even consider to have the authority or proclamation to have the final say over someone's choices and decisions. I can only bring clarity and joy to those who have a listening ear of what I've learned while on this amazing journey of understanding me and going thru my experiences. I hope and pray you, the reader will gravitate and absorb whatever works for you. Remember, Fine luxury living is a lifestyle. It's all incorporated with eating, looking and feeling healthy inside and out. Of course, it comes with acquiring the inner things of life for some or to each its own but at the end of the day, live your best healthy life.

www.ingramcontent.com/pod-product-compliance
Lightning Source LLC
Chambersburg PA
CBHW070117300326

41934CB00035B/1545